Essential Oils

Improve the Quality of your Life with Essential Oils for Health, Beauty, Stress, Energy and more!

Table of Contents

Introduction – Where to Start

There are some common safety precautions you should always take when using any essential oil product:

Only use untainted, therapeutic-grade essential oils and follow usage instructions included with the product.

If any rash or irritation is experienced on the skin when using essential oils, apply a vegetable oil (olive oil, for example) to the affected area.

Never use essential oils on the eyes, inside the ear or in an open wound. If you accidentally affect one of these areas, dilute the essential oil with a vegetable oil, NOT water.

Never consume an essential oil internally unless it is labeled as a dietary supplement, and confirmed as safe for consumption.

If you experience severe side effects, discontinue use of the essential oil that is responsible.

Before using essential oil on children, apply a tiny amount on their skin to test for sensitivity. Do not apply any to a child's hand, as they may transport it to their eyes or mouth.

Consult your physician before using essential oils if you are pregnant or taking any long-term medication.

Keep in mind that therapeutic-grade essential oils are potent plant extracts that must be used with reasonable caution. A consultation with an experienced user of essential oils is the best way to gain a good understanding, and can help ensure you have a positive and rewarding first experience of using them yourself. As your own experience grows, you will learn what works and doesn't work for you, and can take on the role yourself of supporting others as they try incorporating essential oils into their lives.

How are Essential Oils Extracted?

There are several methods that are used to successfully extract essential oils from their host plants. The following list gives a brief overview of them:

Steam distillation

This is done by placing the necessary plant parts, chopped or ground into manageable sizes, on a screen inside a large vat. These vats then have steam forced through the plant parts from beneath, which releases the essential oils into the superheated water vapor. As the steam rises it enters cooling tubes at the top, in which it goes back to its liquid state and leaves a layer of the essential oil at the surface. The oil is then separated and readied for sale, and the distilled water is often put to use as hydrosol or 'floral' water.

Hydro Distillation

Similar to steam distillation, this method dips the plant parts into a hot water pool to extract the oils into the steam, before following the same procedure to separate the water from the oils.

Cold pressing

Typically used on peels or skins of citrus fruits to extract their essential oils. The oils are later filtered to remove impurities and prepped for sale. Sometimes further processing is required to eliminate traces of toxins that are known to cause skin irritation. It is generally advised that you don't use cold pressed citrus oils on skin that is likely to be exposed to sunlight, because it can lead to a phototoxic reaction.

Solvent Extraction

By extracting essential oils using solvents, most commonly carbon dioxide (CO_2) the product is what's known as a 'concrete'. After further processing, a concrete leads to an 'absolute' – an end product that often contains the highest possible amount of minute constituents from the host plant because the oils were not exposed to any water during the process.

Infused oils

Often seen as unreliable sources of essential oils because they have been shown to contain a number of contaminates. Infused oils are made by placing the plant material in a fixed oil such as olive or almond, so that the oils mix and become usable.

When purchasing essential oils, check the label of the packaging as it should list the method of extraction. Trustworthy brands are transparent about what their product contains and how it was extracted, and knowing this information before purchasing can ensure you get exactly the right product to fit your needs.

Chapter 1 - Essential Oils for a Strong Immune System

A strong immune system equips your body with the tools it needs to avoid you getting ill, or fight effectively against illness if it does manage to creep up on you! There are certain chronic ailments that can make you more susceptible to other forms of illness, and strengthening your immune system can help to restrict the extent to which this problem affects your life.

Don't make the mistake of thinking all bacteria and germs are your enemy. All of us have a wealth of helpful bacteria on our skin and at various points in our digestive systems; bacteria which we actually need to keep us alive! They are our friends, helping us extract nutrients from our foods and neutralize harmful toxins. The reality is, most bacteria on our skin are harmless. Of course, we sometimes find ourselves exposed to the OTHER type of bacteria. The ones our bodies need to be prepared to fight against. Almost all essential oils will strengthen the immune system; they all possess anti-bacterial, anti-viral and anti-fungal properties to varying degrees and can therefore help the body fight all kinds of infection.

Diffusion

In general, the most effective way of reaping the benefits from essential oils is to diffuse them into the air. This is the origin of the term 'aromatherapy'; the fragrant oils are released into the air to be inhaled for swift absorption into the body. Diffusing immune supportive essential oils every day is a great way to give your immune system a regular 'tune-up'.

The inhalation of essential oils that have been diffused into the air means they go directly to the lungs. From there they are quickly transferred into the bloodstream through the airway-capillary system, allowing the molecules of the oils to be carried all around the body to pass on their beneficial qualities to every cell in your body. It takes only a few minutes for the blood to complete a circuit of the entire body, so the essential oils you inhale during aromatherapy will have been spread all over your body in a very short period of time, which is great!

What Other Methods of Assimilation are Good?

Mouthwash

Gargling with a liquid, as you would with a mouthwash, is almost as good as inhalation through aromatherapy. The mucus membranes in your mouth are very receptive, and will quickly absorb the essential oils straight into your bloodstream as the capillaries in the lungs do. There will also be the added factor of any lingering vapor in your mouth from the oils being inhaled to the lungs, further increasing your body's assimilation of the oils.

When using an essential oil mouth wash, it is important you don't actually swallow the mixture; simply swish it around the inside of your mouth, then spit it back out. You will only need to use a small drop per ounce of water used for this rinse to be effective. Essential oils are very potent, and the 'heat' of putting too much in your mouth at once may leave you hoping you'll never make that mistake again!

Inhalation is still the preferred method of absorbing essential oils, so you should really only use the mouthwash method if you can't use the inhalation method for any reason, or if you have mouth sores or a sore throat on a particular day. Stick to the number one method as much as possible to get the best results.

Massage Oils

Essentials oils can be effective as part of a massage rub or blend. The absorption process will be slower, happening over a period of several hours as it passes through the skin. Some call this a 'time released' method of essential oil therapy. The skin is the largest organ of the human body, and it will allow some essential oil constituents to pass through its layers into the bloodstream. The oils should be applied as part of carrier lotions to minimize the risk of sensitive skin reactions. Some of the constituents of essential oils are very strong and can cause damage to skin if used in an undiluted form.

A massage can be an incredibly relaxing and fulfilling experience, and with the careful inclusion of essential oils in the massage lotion we can experience further benefits for hours afterwards as the oils continue to pass into the bloodstream.

So, which Essential Oils Strengthen the Immune System?

The first group of essential oils to take note of is the ones that are most commonly associated with increasing activity in some of the mechanisms of the immune system. This group consists of:

Oregano	Eucalyptus Globulus
Sage	Cinnamon Leaf
Bay Laurel	Frankincense

The oils in this group are known to be fairly potent, and it is thus suggested that they be used only when you have been exposed to viruses or other disease-causing organisms.

The second group to consider is the oils that are believed to help strengthen your immune system during periods where you have not actually been exposed to a disease-causing organism. They are said to keep the production of white blood cells in the body at a high level. They include:

Lavender	Bergamot
Myrrh	Sandalwood
Thyme – linalool and vetiver	Roman Chamomile
Pine Needle	Tea Tree
Lemon	

For fighting the damaging effects of being highly **stressed or anxious** – conditions often overlooked when considering the issue of fighting ill health – the recommended essential oils are:

Geranium	Rosemary
Lavender	Tea Tree

These oils are relatively gentle and thus suitable for daily use. You could diffuse them or blends that incorporate them for a pleasant way to help ease stress and keep your body free from its draining effects.

Can I try Ingesting the Oils?

Contrary to the alarming claims of some companies, it is never recommended that you attempt to use essential oils by ingesting them. The oils are potent, concentrated chemicals that could damage the lining of your esophagus and stomach if consumed, either in diluted or undiluted form. They could also do harm to the liver, kidneys and intestinal tract as they continue the journey through your digestive system!

And even without the potential harm you could do to yourself, the truth is that the composition of your stomach pretty much negates the positive effects an essential oil should give you. Your stomach acid will break down some of the constituents of the oil, and what survives that process can harm much of the friendly bacteria in your intestines as it passes through. As a rule, you should only ingest essential oils as capsules or diluted with something else if that was prescribed by a physician. Otherwise, avoid ingesting them at all costs; utilize one of the approved methods of absorbing essential oils into the body to reap their benefits.

What Else do I Need to Know?

Essential oils can only help build the strength of your immune system if you diffuse them on a regular basis over time. Without having done so, you will find that you are more susceptible to common ailments like the common cold or influenza. Of course, essential oils can't grant you immunity to such things, but they can restrict the severity of them when they do strike, and reduce your chances of contracting them in the first place. Begin your treatment by diffusing any of the listed essential oils n a daily basis.

It's not necessary to diffuse a huge amount of your chosen essential oils each day; a few drops in the air during the evening hours should have the desired effect, and repel any bacteria or viruses you may have taken on board during the day.

Don't expect essential oils to function as a substitute for a healthy lifestyle; they should actually be just one component of healthy living. Ensure that you get 7-8 hours of sleep per night, and maintain solid eating and exercise regimens. Failure to adhere to these simple practices will have a negative effect on your immune system. When those times creep up on you when you're stressed, overworked and losing sleep, try to keep up your essential oil diffusion to give your tired body a little boost in fighting illness.

The list included in this chapter suggests some of the essential oils with the best reported results for boosting the immune system, but all essential oils are said to have some value for strengthening it. It is always good practice to diffuse essential oils regularly, because they all have positive properties that will have you looking and feeling better than ever!

Chapter 2 - Aromatherapy

We kept mentioning the term 'Aromatherapy' in chapter 1; undoubtedly it is a word you have heard before, and you probably now realize that it is intrinsically linked with the use of essential oils. There are a number of conventions and theories relating to how Aromatherapy benefits the human body and mind, and the most effective ways to make use of it. If you haven't started using Aromatherapy yet, read on!

The wonderful thing about Aromatherapy is that it is a gift that comes purely from nature, it's very easy to use and it doesn't result in any of the unpleasant side effects that artificial medicines and drugs invariably cause. For the most part they have a beautiful scent, and are safe to use for all members of the family of handled correctly.

So, what's stopping you from getting started right away!? Perhaps you simply don't know where to begin. Most Aromatherapy faithful will always have the foundation of a basic set of essential oils to build upon. The most common introductory oil is Lavender – sometimes known as the 'Mother' of essential oils. It is so called because it essentially possesses qualities to help with all aspects, to varying degrees, of a person's mental and physical wellness. It also has one of the most pleasant aromas.

When searching for Lavender essential oil products, look for the name *Lavendula Angustifolia*; the botanical name for what we call the lavender plant. The factor that most effects the quality of the Lavender oil is its country of origin. Bulgaria and France are known to have good natural conditions for cultivating lavender plants, so it is often recommended that you acquire essential oils sourced from these countries.

Some additional essential oils you may want to include in your basic selection are:

Eucalyptus   *Lemon*

Tea Tree   *Peppermint*

These four are known to have properties that heal many ailments and aid with a variety of issues related to wellness.

As you become more of an established user of essential oils, you may want to add:

Grapefruit	*Rosemary*
Clary Sage	*Ylang-Ylang*

One of the defining principles of Aromatherapy is that you will be inhaling the fragrant oils as they are diffused into the air. Doing so will require that you have some kind of instrument that you can place the oil in so that it diffuses; we call this instrument a diffuser. For your beginning efforts, there is no need to purchase a fancy diffuser. In fact, a simple cotton ball in a glass bowl will suffice! Simply pour a few drops onto the cotton ball, then relax and enjoy the wonderful fragrance.

Don't forget that it is never advised to rub essential oils directly into the skin, unless they have been suitably diluted. The term for an undiluted sample of an essential oil is *'neat'*. Owing to the likelihood that there may be skin sensitivities or allergic reactions to neat essential oils applied directly to the skin, we instead apply it via a *'carrier'*.

Carriers can be creams, lotions, water or a *'fixed'* oil that lacks any skin irritants. There are many options among these to choose from, each with their own benefits for different skin types. Once you have selected the right one for you, the application to your skin is generally done through massage. The most common fixed oils to dilute with are:

Sweet Almond	*Grapeseed Oil*
Jojoba	*Fractionated Coconut*

You might like to consider getting yourself an Aromatherapy recipe book when you begin, so that you can learn some of the most potent blends and methods of dilution. This will give you the most positive early experiences for essential oils, and encourage you to persevere and reap the maximum benefits they have to offer.

As you proceed in learning and experiencing the wonders of essential oils, you will discover that in addition to their ongoing enriching qualities from everyday use, some of them possess more specific functions for helping out when you are feeling unwell, stressed, depressed, bloated, or any other unpleasant situation relating to wellbeing that could arise.

How do I Choose the Right Diffuser for Me?

This is an important question for anyone who is seriously thinking about incorporating essential oils into their daily lives. While all diffusers do, of course, work, there are a number of factors to consider when searching for the best diffuser to meet your personal needs. Here is a brief list of basic questions to consider when making your choice:

Is the diffuser for you or a family member? What ages are the people involved? Are there pets around?

Will you be using it in the house, for an entire office or just on your personal desk?

Are you trying to treat a specific ailment such as a cold, or are you seeking help with emotional problems?

Do you only want to diffuse the scent for treatment, or would you prefer to create an ambience?

What size is the room? How high are the ceilings? Do lots of people come in and out, or is it a more private area?

The consideration of your motivation and the impact that will be made by external factors yields a wide range of questions for you to address. But you will likely find that one of the most pivotal factors is that of your own olfactory system; the physiological system that makes up your sense of smell.

As highly advanced natural creatures, human beings actually rely far more on our sense of smell than you might think. As with so many animals, we use our nose to help with a huge list of tasks that often require its use in combination with other sensory systems. It is part of our primal nature, a deep-rooted component of how we, as animals, experience the world we live in. It can help us to find food and water, but it also protects us against substances, organisms and situations that could harm our survival; through scent, we can detect the presence of predators, fire, or contaminated food.

The strange thing about our olfactory system is that it can sometimes enter a state known as 'olfactory fatigue', in which your sense of smell basically shuts down, for lack of a better phrase. If you've ever been in the presence of a distinctive smell for a long period of time, you may have noticed that after a while you can no longer smell it. This is because your olfactory system has desensitized itself to that smell, due to you learning that it is not a threat to you. Your sense of smell will filter out that perception in favor of looking out for other smells that may potentially pose a threat to you.

This state is detrimental to the process of Aromatherapy, and so selecting the right diffuser can come down to finding one that minimizes your chances of entering olfactory fatigue.

Types of Diffusers

Electric Lighting Oil and Tart warmers: these are great for providing some beautiful ambience lighting, and are an effective method of subtly diffusing essential oils over an extended period of time.

Atomizers or Nebulizers: These use a small pump and some specially designed glass to scatter the essential oil molecules into the air as a fine mist. They should only be used for short periods. The mist of essential oils clouds the area quite quickly, and if this is allowed to continue for more than 7-10 minutes, you can end up with an excessive concentration of essential oils in the air, which can render them ineffective and make the experience far less pleasant for you. The exception to this is when a high concentration of an essential oil is required – say, when treating n ailment – in which case an atomizer is probably the best diffuser to use.

In a large room, an atomizer is the best method for diffusing essential oils to a sufficient extent to cover the entire room. They are powerful diffusers, pumping their mist into the air quite quickly. Many come with a timer to ensure you don't oversaturate a room.

Some diffusers use **tea light candles** under a bowl of water or soy wax tart. These gently release the vapors into the air, but can become very hot over time so make sure you cool the bowl intermittently to avoid heat damage.

There are some very simplistic diffusers that require you to merely place a few drops of essential oil on a surface usually made from **Terra Cotta**. These diffusers disperse the essential oils very slowly.

Chapter 3 - Essential Oils for Energy

We all know that feeling when all your vigor and enthusiasm is eaten away by being overworked, stressed and short of some much-needed sleep! If only you could add a few more hours onto the day to give you some much needed rest so that every other activity would feel like less of a chore! Fatigue is something that many people finds holds them back from achieving their goals. So much to do, so little time, sometimes the things we want to do for our own self-improvement fall by the wayside because our energy is sucked dry as we labor through the things we 'have to do'.

Well, before you turn to excessive coffee drinking, you may want to consider the power of essential oils to rejuvenate and reinvigorate! By incorporating them into your life, you may get back some of that energy, productivity and zest for life that you long for.

Before you start jumping for joy, do be advised that if your fatigue is due to an underlying medical condition, essential oils may only offer short term relief; you will need to keep to your doctor's orders to treat your condition for the long term. But, if it's not caused by a sleep disorder or illness, it could be caused by any or all of the following:

Physical exertion   *Depression*

Hormonal imbalances   *Low blood pressure*

Nutrition   *Stress*

There are many other potential causes of fatigue that can push it to become an obstacle to you fulfilling your productive potential. If you cannot pinpoint a cause for your fatigue, please see your doctor and ask advice on what could be at the heart of it. It could be that you have an underactive thyroid, or nearing an adrenal gland burnout. These are medical conditions that require swift attention, and although essential oils can be used to complement therapy they are not sufficient to treat such conditions by themselves.

Additionally, if you want to maximize your energy levels you should look to eat a healthy diet, exercise regularly, give yourself some regular 'downtime' and get plenty of good-quality sleep!

So which Essential Oils will Help with my Energy Levels?

The most frequently used group of essential oils for boosting energy are the stimulating *Citrus Oils*. These include:

Lemon	*Grapefruit*
Orange	*Bergamot*
Petitgrain	*Neroli*

There is also anecdotal evidence of Spearmint and Peppermint having beneficial effects on energy levels.

During a period where you are fighting the effects of fatigue, you should go all out to pamper yourself. In the morning, take a luxurious aromatherapy bath or shower to breathe life into you for the day. Keep inhaling your stimulating oils and blends throughout the day as you go about your business. Switch to relaxing blends after 6:00pm so that you can wind down, relax and gradually sink into a good night's sleep.

Proven Essential Oil Blends for Relieving Fatigue

The following recipes are for blends that you can implement as great early-morning or after-lunch pick-me-ups:

Energy Boosting Blend

Ginger - 1 drop	*Elemi* - 6 drops
Basil - 3 drops	*Rosemary* - 8 drops
Peppermint - 4 drops	

Blend the ingredients in a small bottle, then add to a diffuser or smell from an inhaler.

Adrenal Gland Help

Peppermint - 1 drop

Cedarwood - 2 drops

Spruce needle - 5 drops

Stimulating Personal Fatigue Relief Blend

Jojoba -1-2 Tablespoons	*Vetiver* - 1 drop
Palmarosa - 1 drop	*Coriander* - 2 drops
Helichrysum - 1 drop	*Clary Sage* - 2 drops
Jasmine - 1 drop	*Orange* - 3 drops

Blend all the essential oils first, then add to the *Jojoba*. Apply the result as you would a perfume, or inhale it from an inhaler.

Alternatively, you can always look in stores for special, pre-prepared blends of essential oils that target fatigue, or indeed any other physical or mental issues. If you don't fancy blending your oils yourself, these are a terrific alternative that are easy to find wherever you purchase your essential oils from.

Keep in mind that short term fatigue is generally an indicator that you need to give yourself more quality rest, but long term fatigue or actual exhaustion can indicate that there is a more urgent medical problem at the heart of it. If your fatigue symptoms cause you any genuine concern, always seek advice from a physician to determine whether there is an underlying condition to blame.

Chapter 4 – Essential Oils for Healing

There are a number of ways our bodies can become damaged. Having accidents or having to undergo surgery can leave you temporarily disabled and in considerate discomfort as you wait for your body to heal. Many people find the scars they are left with unsightly, making them feel self-conscious and leading them to seek ways to make the scarring less visible. When a person finds themselves in one of these situations, they might want to ease their pain, accelerate healing, regain feeling in afflicted areas and minimize the prominence of scars. No company or product can guarantee to deliver on any of these goals, but one would hope that some products offer a measure of relief from the suffering they are put through during the healing process. Well, many essential oils are believed to have just the healing properties you might be looking for!

The capacity to heal wounds can be accelerated by essential oils with the ciatrisant, or 'cell regenerative', property. These oils include:

Helichrysum   *Lavender*

Rose   *Neroli*

Sage   *Niaouli*

Rosemary   *Cistus*

Frankincense

There are over two dozen ciatrisant essential oils, possessing varying degrees of potency for accelerating the healing process. Those in the previous list are the ones that are most commonly used.

Diluted Lavender can be applied around most open wounds. It assists the body in fighting infection, and accelerates healing by promoting the regeneration of new cells. The swifter a wound is able to heal, the less likely it is to leave a scar.

Helichrysum is also very effective if applied around new wounds, particularly when there is also bruising involved. It promotes cell regeneration and also relieves pain by targeting the healing of nerve cells. It has some effect on older wounds or scars, but is most effective on recent wounds.

Applying Essential Oils to Minor Wounds

When a small wound has just been incurred, clean the afflicted area using 2 cups of warm water, each of which has had 5 drops of Lavender and 2-3 drops of Tea Tree added. This will serve to both clean and disinfect the area. If a wound is particularly dirty from debris, you might want to use a mild soap solution for more thorough cleaning. Then repeat the first step for a final rinse.

Applying Essential Oils to Stitched Wounds

If a cut has been severe enough to require stitches for healing, consult your doctor to ensure they have no objection to you applying diluted Lavender to the site. Some doctors will prefer you wait until the stitches are removed; in this case, ask if the doctor objects to the proposal of applying your essential oils around the wound's perimeter without actually touching the stitches themselves.

Remember there are numerous essential oils constituents which can be absorbed by the skin to enter blood vessels and be transported around the body. Even if you are unable to apply healing oils directly onto the affected area, you can still benefit from their healing properties. The cells that benefit from those healing properties will still be supplied with them through the bloodstream.

Treating Scars

Sage and Neroli are known to play a positive role in preventing and minimizing scarring.

Once a cut has been sealed shut by the body's healing, you can begin to apply essential oil blends known for their abilities to reduce scarring. It is important that you don't peel off any scabs. Apply your blend over the scab and the skin surrounding it. Any damage you do to the scab itself carries a large risk of causing a scar, so be careful as you interfere with the region.

You can concoct a powerful blend by mixing 10 drops of Helichrysum into 1 ounce of Rosehipseed oil, which you can apply to a wound once or twice per day to accelerate healing. Aromatherapy theory states that this blend helps accelerate slow-healing wounds and prevent keloid formation; by accelerating the healing, this blend reduces the risk of being left with scarring from a wound.

If you have old scars, and would like to reduce their prominence on the skin, you will need to be prepared to have a little patience and a lot of perseverance. It will require a daily treatment using any of the oils in our original list, but it can take as much as 3 to 6 months for you to even begin to notice any results. Commitment and consistency are the most challenging requirements if you want to succeed in reducing old scars.

Case Study

A female patient underwent a surgery called abdominoplasty (commonly known as a 'tummy tuck'). Whilst healing from the surgery, she used a mixture of Rosehipseed Oil and Hazelnut Oil – two very skin nourishing carrier oils – with Lavender, Helichrysum, Neroli and Sage. When the wound had fully healed, the 20-inch incision line was barely visible. In fact, when the patient was not 'tanned' from the sun, the presence of the scar was almost impossible to see! This was a powerful blend, and the results she achieved speak for themselves.

She didn't begin applying her blend until all the sutures had been removed from the area – this actually delayed her in starting the scarring treatment for a whopping 3 weeks! She did apply diluted Lavender around the perimeter of the large sutured region reducing the inflammation and itching that usually accompanies the healing process. As a result, she continued applying the diluted Lavender once the stitches came out, but she still maintains that had she been able to begin the scarring treatment sooner, she would have achieved even better results. After 6 months of commitment to the cause, she was fully healed and the scarring was all but invisible.

When healing from a sizeable wound or surgical incision, you will experience a variety of unusual sensations as the affected region develops. These include:

Numbness

Inability to distinguish between hot and cold

Sensation of something crawling on the skin

Itchiness

The itchiness is common to the healing process of all cuts and wounds. It is a sign that the body is working to rebuild damaged material; don't scratch the area if you can possibly resist it, as you will only make the irritation worse and potentially add to the scarring that will result. Ignore the itch as best you can, and eventually it will fade away.

The odd feelings listed above are all normal sensations brought about by the nerve cells regenerating and 'waking up'. The wound may have caused nerve endings in the area to be completely severed, and it takes a very long time for this to fully regenerate. The result is that you may experience some of those odd sensations for years after the wound has healed!

To help the body continue the cellular regeneration that will eventually eliminate those sensations, you can keep using Helichrysum or the previously described scar treatment blend on a daily basis. Doing so can help your body to heal the damaged area to a far greater degree than it could if you didn't give it the extra support.

Everyone's experience of the healing process will be different, but the suggestions in this chapter are all-natural, inexpensive actions you can take to alleviate unpleasant feelings, accelerate the body's own healing capabilities, and hopefully minimize any resulting scarring. If you choose to take up the essential oil strategies, remember to use the right carrier oils and to be consistent and committed to your treatment. Only then will you see the results you desire! Everyone will heal and react differently but the suggestions here are an all-natural method and very inexpensive thing to do. So, if you wish to give them a try, remember essential oils and some nourishing carrier oils are very effective at helping you lighten those awful scars!

Scarring and Young Children

Young children, particularly those under 5, fall over frequently. Sometimes these falls result in cuts, and in certain areas – chin, eyebrow, etc – where there is little between the skin's surface and the bone, these cuts can leave scars. If your young child has been cut in one of these areas, consult a physician to check if they are happy for you to apply a scar lightening blend.

For children less than 2 years old, there is always the chance that they might rub the area where you apply the blend and then rub their eyes or mouth. In this case it is recommended that you only use rosehip seed oil, again with the permission of a doctor. This can be applied several times a day to promote healing and fight scarring.

Chapter 5 – Essential Oils for Weight Loss

Essential oils are not a shortcut to achieving your weight loss goals. But if you incorporate them into your lifestyle, they can be the final boost your body needs to push past your next milestone and go on to eventually meet your ideal weight. When addressing any issue relating to our health, we must take a holistic approach; one which accounts for all the factors that can affect the way our body functions. This includes digestive performance, stress levels, diet and exercise, habits and lifestyle, and more serious considerations such as underlying medical conditions, emotional turmoil and the like. Basically, in order to achieve our health and wellness goals, we must take an honest look at every component of our lives that will affect them, and aim to make a holistic effort to improve. The mistake many people make when trying to lose weight is only factoring in some of those considerations, leading to frustration when progress is slow, or non-existent!

There are a number of weight loss supplements on the market, usually created through artificial methods and containing various sugars and stimulants like caffeine. The essential oils you can use to assist in weight loss contain nothing artificial, and do not cause any side effects (except perhaps skin irritation in exceptional cases). As part of a holistic approach, essential oils can assist you in reaching your target weight in an all-natural, stress-free way.

The great thing about the essential oils we generally use for metabolic (weight loss) blends is that they also have superb properties for improving your emotional state. These blends can have a strong effect on your psychological self-image; you will be more able to feel comfortable in your own skin, with a positive body image and acceptance of who you naturally are. This will help to overcome the problem of setting yourself unnecessary weight loss goals; having a positive emotional framework will reduce a person's insecurities. The goal in adding essential oils to your weight loss strategy is to find a spiritual connection with your body, so that the full spectrum of mind, body and spirit are aligned! These are benefits that every person could be enriched by.

The Best Essential Oils for Weight Loss

Using essential oils singularly can have some effect, but it is through the use of the most potent blends that you will experience the maximum benefits those oils have to offer. Aim to purchase therapeutic grade essential oils for your blends, as these will contain the purest and most powerful oils. The following list contains the individual essential oils that are used in the most popular weight loss blends:

Lemon: Known for its detoxifying uses, this oil can increase energy levels and is said to fight intestinal parasites and numerous digestive maladies. It is also believed to positively influence one's self-judgment and self-approval.

Grapefruit: This oil has worked wonders for people in tackling cellulite, reducing appetite and toning the body, as well as lowering stress and promoting positive thinking. It is often used as a complementary method in treating eating disorders and improving a person's body image.

Cinnamon: It is said that cinnamon can act as a catalyst for other weight-loss-focused essential oils. It can also have an impact in maintaining healthy insulin levels, improving digestion and circulation and even increasing libido. Psychologically it encourages greater love for one's self, allowing you to feel more free and comfortable.

Ginger: Ginger has a great reputation for its positive influence on digestive issues. Additionally, it can boost energy levels, warm the body and stimulate increased activity in the body's self-sustaining systems. It can also evoke a strong sense of empowerment, boosting one's confidence and motivation when taking on challenges such as weight loss goals!

Peppermint: This oil is renowned for its positive effects on a wide range of digestive issues, and it is also a stimulant for intellectual activity! It is said to repress strong negative emotional states like depression, and promote optimism and positivity in the mind and spirit.

Now, there is clearly a spectacular array of desirable properties spread throughout this selection of essential oils. The key to harnessing their power is in concocting the perfect blends that combine these properties in a complementary way. Remember, although it is possible that you might experience weight loss results just by using an essential oil blend, the most likely way to experience change is by incorporating the blend into your holistic approach to change.

Precautions: Citrus oils can cause increased sensitivity to the sun's rays. If you're applying a blend to the skin, do so at night within at least 12 hours before you next expose yourself to sunlight. If you are pregnant or nursing, consult a doctor before beginning to use weight loss blends. Always test how a blend affects skin sensitivity, and apply in areas that will remain covered if possible. Remember that overuse of any essential oil can cause skin irritation, and they must be kept out of the eyes, ears and nose. The quality of the oils you use will determine their effectiveness, and only use them in the ways directed by the maker of an essential oil.

Weight Loss Blend Recipes

Weight Loss Citrus Blend

30 drops **Grapefruit**

4 drops **Lemon**

1 drop **Ylang-Ylang**

Weight Loss Mint Blend

20 drops **Peppermint**

10 drops **Bergamot**

4 drops **Spearmint**

1 drop **Ylang-Ylang**

Weight Loss Herbal Blend

15 drops **Basil**

15 drops **Marjoram**

1 drop **Oregano**

1 drop **Thyme**

How to Consume your Weight Loss Blends

Listed below are some suggestions, from recognized sources in the field of aromatic study, for how you can apply your chosen blend to tackle different issues relating to weight loss. Use them as guidelines, or as inspiration to come up with your own methods. See what works for you and your body.

Appetite Reduction

Add 2-3 drops of your weight loss blend to every drink of water you have throughout the day. Inhaling from the bottle is also acceptable.

Repress Cravings

Add 1 drop of your weight loss blend to an ounce of water and swallow, or inhale from the bottle if you prefer.

Boost Metabolism

Add 1-2 drops of your blend into every glass of water you drink, or massage it into the reflex points of your feet.

Cellulite Reduction

Massage 1-2 drops of your blend into the affected area every day.

Tackling Obesity

Add 1-2 drops of your blend to every glass of water you consume.

Reduce Sugar Cravings

Add 1 drop of your blend to an ounce of water 3 times per day. Or, inhale from the bottle as required.

Managing Overeating

Add 1-2 drops to a glass of water before you eat.

Boost Energy

Diffuse, add 1-2 drops to water, or massage into soles of feet every day.

Mental Stimulation

Use a diffuser to inhale during periods of fatigue or stress.

Calming/Relaxation

Inhale your blend from the bottle as required.

Blood Sugar Regulation

Rub several drops of your blend into the soles of the feet. Do this 1-2 times per day. Adding 1-2 drops to drinking water is also acceptable.

Circulation

Rub several drops of your blend into the chest around the heart region. Alternatively, rub several drops each day into any region where circulation is a concern.

Detox
Add a few drops to every drink of water, or rub into the reflex points of the feet.

Improve Digestion

Add several drops to a glass of water each day, or rub 2 drops into your abdomen.

Increase Self-Worth/Develop Self-Confidence/Feel Uplifted

Diffuse or inhale from the bottle periodically throughout the day. Alternatively, try massaging 1-2 drops into the solar plexus region of your abdomen.

Chapter 6 – Essential Oils for Beauty

The beauty industry has come to something of a crossroads.

More than ever before, we have the ability to use miraculous ingredients and techniques to fight the signs of ageing and correct what we see as 'imperfections' or 'flaws'. However, the exciting potential of such promising 'cosmeceuticals' and non-invasive procedures does not come without a significant concern regarding the long-term effects. In a nutshell, many people are worried that the short-term benefits to one's appearance that science's wonders offer may not be worth the potential risk they pose for the long term. The result is that there has been an increase in the number of people turning to organic, natural alternatives that have been tried and tested for years – some even centuries!

One of the figureheads of organic beauty treatments is an aromatherapy guru named Daniele Ryman. She has been practicing aromatherapy for over four decades, and firmly believes in the anti-ageing properties of essential oils. She was mentored by the doyenne of aromatherapy Marguerite Maury. Recalling one of her early experiences with essential oils, Daniele told the following story:

"Marguerite first suggested aromatherapy to me when I complained about a wrinkly I had noticed near my eye at the age of 22. She made me a special blend, which I still have the recipe for. It was geranium, eucalyptus, neroli and rose mixed in a carrier of hazelnut, avocado and almond. It smelt wonderful and was so helpful that I instantly became hooked."

It is Daniele's expertise that we will draw upon for this chapter, presenting you with 10 of her most powerful recipes for head-to-toe beauty treatment done the organic way:

Hair – Ylang-Ylang Hair Loss Remedy

Any type of hair loss can be absolutely devastating. It could be a result of cancer treatment, stress or hormone imbalances. Hair treatments using ylang-ylang have been used effectively since way back in the 19th century, and the following recipe is based on a trusted treatment called Macassar. Before applying, tip your head forwards and brush your hair, continuing to do so until you can feel your scalp becoming warm.

6 drops of **ylang-ylang**	1 capsule **evening primrose oil**
1 capsule **borage oil**	1 x 50ml bottle

Mix the oils and shake extensively. Massage the blend into your scalp around one hour before shampooing. Do this 2-3 times per month. You can also add a few drops of the blend to a mild shampoo; just make sure you shake well before applying.

Face – Parsley Facial Cleanser

On the cheeks and around the eyes, broken capillaries can be quite prominent. The best preventative measure for these is to avoid overly hot showers or baths, hot facials, exposure to bright sunlight and excessive alcohol, as these things can cause capillaries to dilate. Try to consume lots of Vitamin C and Rutin (which comes from citrus fruits). Both of these assist in strengthening the walls of blood vessels.

The essential oils that are known to be effective in reducing the appearance of broken capillaries are parsley, chamomile, orange and violet leaves.

30ml rose **masqueta oil**

10ml **argan oil**

2 capsules **borage oil**

2 capsules **wheatgerm oil**

6 drops of **parsley**

2 drops of **chamomile/violet leaves/orange**

1 x 50ml bottle

Mix the blend in the bottle and gently rub it into the face after cleansing in the morning. Leave for 10 minutes, then gently remove any remaining oil with a tissue or baby wipe. This blend will keep for 2-3 months.

Eyes – Gentle Oil Blend

Bags under the eyes are caused by lack of sleep, too much alcohol and smoking, and sometimes by allergies. The skin around the eyes is extremely delicate, and sometimes the moisturizing creams we think should help are actually contributing to the problem. Instead, try using the following light blend.

1/2 **cucumber**, liquidized

1 capsule **wheatgerm oil**

50ml herbal infusion - **fennel, comfrey, marigold** or **parsley**

Concoct this infusion using a teaspoon of your selected herb and 50ml of boiled water. Allow this mixture to cool, strain it, then stir in the liquidized cucumber and the wheatgerm.

Using your fingertip, gently apply the gel to the area around your eye. It will reduce puffiness and wrinkles, and increase circulation to make skin appear more vibrant. Keep the blend refrigerated and use it up within 3 days.

Lips – Natural Balm

It is no secret that lip enhancement is a sought-after goal in beauty. People often opt for injections and surgical intervention to get the luscious lips they desire.

The following natural lip balm should be rubbed into your lips twice a day, and will give you that fuller pout you desire in no time.

10ml **jojoba oil**	2 capsules **wheatgerm oil**
5ml **castor oil**	1 x 50ml bottle
5ml **argan oil**	

Shake the blend together in the bottle and apply carefully to your lips, gently rubbing it in with your fingertips. Massage into the skin around the mouth as well in a clockwise motion. When you have covered the entire area, leave it to be absorbed for a few minutes then remove the surplus with a tissue. Repeat this process twice a day, and keep the blend refrigerated for up to 1 month.

Neck – Toning Massage Oil Blend

The area around the jaw line and neck can become a very obvious indicator of ageing. Essential oil massages to this region can work wonders in fighting those signs of ageing! The following blend should be massaged into the neck and jaw line in upward movements that gently lift, pinch and hold your skin in order to tighten and tone the area.

10ml **jojoba oil**	10 drops of **sandalwood**
8ml **avocado oil**	5 drops of **bois de rose**
2 capsules **borage oil**	2 drops of **petit grain** OR **orange**
4 capsules **wheatgerm oil**	1 x 50ml bottle

Shake the ingredients together in the bottle. Before applying, place a hot flannel over the region for several minutes to open the pores and help with penetration. Apply the blend using the massage technique described above every night; the recipe should provide enough of the blend for 2-3 weeks. Keep it refrigerated, and repeat the entire process 2-3 times a year.

Breasts – Aromatic Vinegar Lotion

You can create a lotion that is very effective in firming connective tissue around the breasts. It is easy to make, and can help to maintain the shape and suppleness of the breasts. You can use the essential oils rose, bois de rose, ylang-ylang, peppermint or lavender; the choice is yours.

15 drops of your chosen essential oil

1/2 liter **cider** or **white wine** vinegar

3/4 liter **boiled cold water**

1 x 2-litre bottle

Put the cider or white vinegar into the bottle first, then your chosen essential oil. Leave this mixture in a dark place for 2 weeks, then add the water to the blend. Use cotton wool to apply the lotion using circular motions to each breast. Repeat the process several times in one sitting, then allow the skin to dry. Use this preparation daily for 2 months.

Arms – Massage Oil for the Upper Arms

The skin on the upper arms can begin to sag with age, and they are a body part that is often on show when we go out. Cardiovascular exercise such as walking, running or swimming can help tone and firm the upper arms, and gently massaging upwards with the following blend will encourage lymphatic drainage and fight droopage and cellulite.

45ml **jojoba oil**

10ml rose **masqueta oil**

1 capsule **wheatgerm oil**

1 capsule **evening primrose oil**

3 drops of **rose** OR **jasmine**

5 drops of **lavender**

4 drops of **bois de rose** OR **lemon**

1 x 100ml bottle

Mix the blend in the bottle. After bathing or showering, massage the oil into the triceps muscle region, starting at the elbow and moving upwards. This blend will keep for up to 2 months.

Hands – Fading Oil for Age Spots

Ageing spots, often known as 'liver spots', can appear from excessive exposure to the sun as well as being a sign of ageing. The following massage oil can help reduce their appearance.

15ml **almond oil**	10 drops of **lavender**
15ml **argan oil**	2 drops of **rose**
1 capsule **wheatgerm oil**	1 x 50ml bottle
2 capsules **evening primrose oil**	

Mix together in the bottle and shake well. Massage the oil into the hands until fully absorbed every evening. The blend will keep for up to 2 months, so use it until it is finished.

Buttocks – Cellulite Massage Oil

Around 90% of women are affected by cellulite, which is often brought on by hormonal changes involving estrogen levels. High estrogen encourages greater fluid retention in the body, which in turn clumps the fat cells together and causes an 'orange peel' appearance at the surface of the skin in some areas. Most commonly it affects the buttocks and hamstring regions, and a holistic approach of diet, exercise, detox baths and body brushing is encouraged to maximize your fight against it. The following massage oil will also help, using guarana to activate circulation and stimulate increased blood flow.

10ml **aloe vera juice**	5 drops of **thyme** OR **fennel**
20ml **almond oil**	6 drops of **rose**
60ml **grapeseed oil**	10 drops of **lemon, grapefruit** OR **orange**
10ml **guarana tea**	
2 capsules **wheatgerm oil**	10 drops of **cypress** OR **violet leaves**
1 capsule **borage oil**	1 x 100ml bottle

Pour all ingredients into the bottle and shake thoroughly. This oil will need to sit on the surface of the skin for several minutes before you massage it in. Massage into affected areas once per day.

Note: Shake the bottle well before every application, as the contents of the blend will separate over time.

Stored in a cool, dark place this blend will keep for 3-4 weeks.

Legs – Vitamin-Rich Massage Lotion

Interruptions of the blood flow in certain regions can cause those dreaded varicose veins. People who stand a lot are more susceptible to them, as are those who either don't exercise, or exercise too strenuously! They can also be the result of genetics.

The following blend is effective in preventing varicose veins, but can also help minimize their appearance of you already have them. The ingredients are rich in Vitamin C and rutin, which will help strengthen the walls of capillaries. The geranium will promote good circulation, and the citrus oils can be beneficial to the vascular system as a whole. The aroma is also very uplifting.

Note that, to avoid varicose veins, you are advised to eat lots of fruit, avoid very heavy lifting and not take too many hot baths!

50ml **soya oil**	1 drop of **lemon**
1 capsule **wheatgerm oil**	1 drop of **orange**
2 drops of **geranium**	1 x 50ml bottle
2 drops of **grapefruit**	

Shake the ingredients well in the bottle. Rub the oil very gently into the legs using upward motions, starting at the feet and finishing at the thighs. Repeat this process daily, and the blend should keep for 2-3 months.

Conclusion

It is not the claim of this book that essential oils are an all-purpose remedy that will magically transform your life into one of beauty, good health and peace of mind. The world of complementary and alternative therapies will consistently tell you that in order for its methods to have the greatest impact on your life, you must take a holistic approach to bringing about change. Essential oils are but one component of this holistic method, and their successful use requires commitment and discipline for the long term.

That being said, the correct use of essential oils can yield very positive results in the areas covered in this book. There are a number of ways they can be incorporated into your lifestyle, and even more theories about the most effective method of consuming them. You will need to experiment and do your own research to find whether the right method for you is to use a diffuser of some kind, or massage oils, or perhaps a mouthwash or even part of a beverage you prepare. Finding what works for you is not just about discovering which method seems to be the most effective, but also which you can most comfortably incorporate into your lifestyle to ensure it stays with you for the long term.

Some people enjoy the ambience aromatherapy diffusers can bring, and use them to complement meditation or exercises such as yoga or Pilates. Others enjoy the 'spa'-type treatment of a massage and perhaps using oils while bathing. The general theme is that they can bring about a sense of relaxation and positivity, and universally promote the ideal of taking some time out to look after yourself. This is a great message for anyone to get behind; one which we could all benefit from as we seek to improve our quality of life.

All essential oils are said to possess qualities that can boost the immune system. Strengthening that fundamental process of your body will enable you to experience natural improvements in your external and internal self. Your skin will be softer and fresher, you will find it easier to lose weight and eat right. Exercise will be easier, and recovery times will be shorter. As a result, your confidence and self-esteem will grow, making you stronger and more positive psychologically. All these attributes can be nurtured even further by utilizing the blends and suggestions in this book, and other essential oil methods you research for yourself.

The foundation you will establish by incorporating essential oils into your life will give you a platform to work on the aspects of yourself that you feel you want to improve. As long as you adhere to the guidelines for safe and proper use, there is no negative side to using them, and as you become more learned and experienced you will find yourself able to identify exactly what you need, and how to make it happen. Essential oils are a way to get back in touch with nature's intentions for our animal selves. Try it for yourself; you'll be glad you did!

www.ingramcontent.com/pod-product-compliance
Lightning Source LLC
Chambersburg PA
CBHW070525290526
45790CB00003B/1304